THE MAGIC OF HUMOR
IN CAREGIVING

Other books by James R. Sherman, Ph.D.

How to Overcome a Bad Back
How to Survive Rejection and Promote Acceptance
Get Set...GO!
Escape to the Gunflint
Stop Procrastinating: Get to Work
Plan Your Work: Work Your Plan
* *Sharpening Your Edge*

In the DO IT! Success Series

Stop Procrastinating–DO IT!
Patience Pays Off
No More Mistakes
Plan for Success
Farewell to Fear
Be a Winner

In the Caregiver Survivor Series

Preventing Caregiver Burnout
Creative Caregiving
Positive Caregiver Attitudes
The Magic of Humor in Caregiving
* *The Caregiver's Guide to Problem Solving*
* *Conquering Caregiver Fears*
* *Strengthening the Caregiver Family*
* *Love, Companionship, and Caregiving*
* *Health Strategies for Active Caregivers*
* *The Caregiver's Need for People*
* *The Caregiver's Planning Guide*
* *Financial Fitness for Caregivers*

* = books in production

THE MAGIC OF HUMOR IN CAREGIVING

James R. Sherman, Ph.D.

Pathway Books

Library of Congress Catalog Card Number
James R. Sherman
The Magic of Humor in Caregiving

International Standard Book Number
0–935538–19–4

Manufactured in the United States of America by Malloy Lithographing, Inc.

Design by Group Design

0 9 8 7 6 5 4 3 2 1

Pathway Books
700 Parkview Terrace
Golden Valley, Minnesota 55416–3439
(612) 377–1521

Dedicated to Caregivers

"The capacity to care is the thing that
gives life its deepest significance and meaning."

PREFACE

This book contains a wealth of ideas about the magic of humor for caregivers like you who want to learn how to live better but have a limited time for reading. Use it as a valuable resource guide. Familiarize yourself with the contents as you go through it for the first time, then come back again and again whenever a need arises. Like any good resource, this book will always provide an easy–to–follow solution or tell you where to go to find one.

Have a pen or pencil handy as you read *The Magic of Humor in Caregiving* and mark the pages that are important to you. Answer the questions that are asked, fill in the lists, and add notes of your own whenever you can expand on a usable idea. Let the book work for you.

Keep in mind that this is a self–help book that is going to make you a better caregiver. It will re–ignite your zest for caregiving and get you feeling good again as long as you keep harvesting the material it contains.

If you can find something to laugh at, no matter how serious your situation is, you'll see caregiving in a new and refreshing way. That doesn't mean you're being disrespectful of your care receiver or the condition that brings you together. Nor does it mean that you have to find humor in everything. It just means you've tried to lighten the impact of one of life's misfortunes and tried to make your situation more enjoyable.

ACKNOWLEDGEMENTS

My wife Merlene has guided me through the complex world of caregiving. She has spent countless hours pulling, pushing, reviewing, editing, and otherwise shaping my thoughts as I wrote these books. It has been said that the supreme test of marriage is when husbands and wives put up wallpaper together. That doesn't stand a candle to writing, editing, designing, printing, and marketing a series of books. I could never in a million years have brought these books to life if it had not been for her help.

Special thanks go to Chris Sherman, our eldest son, editor, and friend. Like his brothers, Eric and Lincoln, he is doing everything he can to bring us into the 21st century.

I would also like to thank Bruce Eaton, Gina Copley, Gretchen Blase and Lori Anderson at Group Design, Brigid Alseth, Edna Ballard, Joan Bowlin, Rev. Dr. Ed Daniel, Audrey De La Martre, Thelma Edwards, Etta Erickson, Lynn Friss Feinberg, Karen Hanauer, Sally Hebson, Phyllis Johnson, Betty Kane, Marilyn Kelly, Art Linkletter, Lindsey McDivitt, Rev. Irven Nelson, Julie Nygren, Pat Peterson, Dr. Loran Pilling, Robert Provost, Jane Royse, Jane and Rev. David Ruhmkorff, Dr. Lawrence Schut, Gail Skoglund, and Elva Walker for their kind words, support, suggestions, and encouragement.

If there are errors in fact, style, format, or whatever, they are mine to bear.

ENDORSEMENTS

Brigid Alseth, President, Minnesota Adult Daycare Association
> *"The lighthearted style of this book will make caregivers sit up, take notice and re–evaluate the humor in their lives."*

Edna L. Ballard, ACSW, Senior Fellow, Duke University Center for the Study of Aging and Human Development
> *"Dr. Sherman's straightforward suggestions on the use of humor in caregiving offer enormous benefits to both caregivers and care receivers. His new look at the relationships between them confirms the fact that neither caregivers nor care receivers must <u>always</u> be serious; humor is a healthy and necessary coping skill."*

Joan Mason Bowlin, Geriatric Nurse Practitioner
> *"The Magic of Humor in Caregiving provides a methodical approach to developing a sense of humor in an occupation that is all too often grim."*

The Reverend Dr. C. Edwin Daniel, United Methodist Minister
> *"Dr. Sherman places not only caregiving but all of life into proper perspective. Caregivers <u>and</u> care receivers will both discover words of wisdom in these words of humor."*

Thelma Edwards, R.N., Director of Program Development, National Stroke Association
> *"The information provided in the Caregiver Survival Series is valuable for both caregivers and stroke survivors as they proceed as 'partners' on the road to recovery. This book, which is enjoyable and easy to read, stresses the importance of laughter and positive humor in coping with day-to-day activities."*

Etta Erickson, Oncology Social Worker, Abbott Northwestern Hospital

" ...offers a host of ideas for introducing the healing element of humor into a stress-filled life. This easy-to-read primer on therapeutic humor invites the discovery of amusement and even joy into the turbulence of caregiving."

Lynn Friss Feinberg, Family Caregiver Alliance

" ...an uplifting and refreshing book, emphasizing the importance of humor and positive coping in caregiving. It will serve as a comfort to many caregivers."

Karen Hanauer, Employee Assistance Counselor, Cargill, Inc.

"Humor is music to the soul. This inspiring book provides an enlightened approach to caregiving with imagination and hope. It's packed with tangible tools and indispensable resources for corporations that are involved with employee eldercare issues."

Phyllis Hahn Johnson, caregiver group facilitator

" ...lifts our spirits and enables us to see the humor in some of the frustrating incidents that face us everyday. I have not found another resource like this."

Lindsey McDivitt, Coordinator, Stroke Education Services, Courage Center

"Dr. Sherman introduces caregivers to the benefits of laughter but also recognizes the darker side of caregiving. Sources of humor and inspirational techniques are presented in a format that makes them available even to caregivers who are feeling overwhelmed."

Rev. Irven Nelson, Lutheran Pastor

" ...a very important contribution to the whole area of caregiving. This book will be a very useful tool for clergy of all denominations and faiths."

Julie Nygren, R.N., Director of Family Services, Alzheimer's Association

> *"...Caring for a loved one with Alzheimer's disease requires unlimited, positive emotional energy. My spirits were lifted after reading* The Magic of Humor in Caregiving; *other caregivers will experience similar feelings."*

Pat Peterson, single working mother and caregiver

> *"The books in the Caregiver Survival Series have been a lifesaver. You get what you need when you need it. They've helped to ease my mind, because I know now that I am not alone. I can't wait to read them all."*

Loran Pilling, M.D., psychiatrist in private practice

> *"Dr. Sherman has captured, in a readable, thought-provoking style, the value of humor in relieving the tensions that naturally occur in caregiving. He gives the caregiver permission to feel anger, fear and sadness without feeling guilty, and then through humor demonstrates the best way to maintain a healthy caregiving relationship."*

Bob Provost, caregiver and Chair, Metropolitan Agency on Aging

> *"The Caregiver Survival Series has given me new insights into my own caregiving this past year. The Magic of Humor in Caregiving is a wonderful resource to assist each of us in our daily challenge."*

Jane Royse, Manager, Alzheimer's Care Center, Minnesota Masonic Home

> *"...a must-read survival guide for every caregiver who has forgotten how to laugh or who no longer finds humor in life's many challenges."*

Jane and Rev. David Ruhmkorff, caregiver and stroke survivor

> *"It takes three things to make a person whole; a goal, a variety of interests and a sense of humor. Dr. Sherman's strategies and solutions definitely confirm this holistic approach to living and caregiving."*

Gail Skoglund, Social Worker, Intergenerational Daycare
  "...clearly demonstrates the importance of humor in caregiving. This book is a valuable, uplifting tool for <u>all</u> caregivers, including professionals. We will definitely use it in our support groups."

Elva D. Walker, Previous Chair, National Council on Aging
  "Without humor, what do you have? I found this book interesting, very timely and an extremely important component of the Caregiver Survival Series."

TABLE OF CONTENTS

THE ESSENCE OF HUMOR

☐ OPENERS

"Good humor is the health of the soul, sadness is its poison."
- Leszczynski Stanislas, 18th century Polish king.

Lou Cook joined a caregiver support group three years after his wife was diagnosed with Alzheimer's disease. At his first meeting, Lou was asked what he thought about caregiving. *"Caregiving,"* he said, *"is a lot like high-school algebra. Every time you get one problem solved, the teacher is waiting to give you another."*

Lou's comment brought chuckles to a group that too often had been dealing with anger and frustration in their daily lives. As the evening went on, other caregivers in the group offered their lighthearted definitions of caregiving. The group finally settled on one comment that best described their feelings. *"Caregiving sometimes feels like a set of fingernails scratching on the blackboard of life."*

Lou thinks his support group saved his life. It didn't make his caregiving tasks any easier, but he was finally able to handle those tasks with a much healthier attitude. Lou felt, like many other caregivers, that the stress and strain of taking care of someone who was physically disabled or mentally impaired was a subject for poets, not humorists. Then, encouraged by his support group, he began to read about the therapeutic effects of humor.

Lou discovered what American humorist Steve Allen has known all along, that *"humor is the essence of humanity."* He sees it as a form of communication that allows him to say things that would be hard to relate otherwise, like using humor to express his frustration. His sense of humor helps him see the beauty of life beyond the hardships of caregiving.

Lou understands the tragedy of Alzheimer's, stroke, cancer, heart disease and the many other ailments that afflict those who need care. But he also recognizes the magic of humor in caregiving, in its availability, applicability and universality. His feelings of anger and frustration haven't disappeared entirely, but they appear far less often. He smiles more frequently, enjoys the company of other people more and can laugh at many of the tender moments that he and Betty have shared over the years.

Lou can find bits of humor everywhere, and he has learned to apply them to every aspect of his life. He shares his humor with other caregivers who are in the same disheartening situation he's in. He touts humor as one of the best tonics caregivers can find to get through a future of uncertainty and apprehension, regardless of their care receiver's affliction. Lou is convinced that of all the strategies caregivers need, a sense of humor is probably the one they need most.

☐　HUMOR IS EVERYWHERE

"From there to here, from here to there, funny things are everywhere."
- Dr. Seuss, American writer and illustrator.

Everybody has a sense of humor, even if it's seldom used. If you haven't energized yours lately, it might be a little rusty and need some polishing. You can increase your laughter capacity and improve your caregiving experience by creating a lifestyle in which humor is a conscious and significant element. That requires desire, courage, hard work, determination and discipline. It also calls for a deep-seated commitment on your part to find happiness in what might otherwise be unhappy circumstances. If you're successful, you'll not only be a better caregiver, you'll be a much healthier one over the long haul.

You have to have a method or procedure to follow and you have to know where you want to go. Because if you don't know where you're going, you'll probably end up someplace else.

The first thing you have to do to enhance your sense of humor is develop your ability to recognize the humorous events that occur around you in everyday situations, including your caregiving experiences.

You have to be able to see and enjoy the funny side of life in and out of caregiving. Sometimes that's awfully hard to do. But having that ability or not having it is one of the biggest differences between those who possess a keen sense of humor and those who do not.

The American humorist Will Rogers had no trouble finding things to laugh about. *"I don't make jokes,"* he said, *"I just watch the government and report the facts."*

You can find humor in your home in the spontaneous and often uninhibited thoughts, sayings and actions of your care receiver. You can find it in all the hilarious antics that are so characteristic of children and grandchildren.

Humor abounds in the workplace, particularly among the miscues and plain ridiculous things that are said and done by employers and employees alike. Can you imagine the horse laughs that followed this notice in the Evergreen State College employee handbook: *"The Equal Pay Act of 1963 requires equal sex for equal work."*

Sometimes the stress of deadlines or the importance of certain caregiving tasks can hide the humor. But then the stress passes and the goof-ups are brought to full bloom and discussed at work, at the dinner table, in support groups or in other less stressful situations.

Much of the best humor is found in the frequently tragic reality of human experience. Here's an example.

When John got off the bus after a two-week trip to the city, the first person he met was his neighbor Bill.
"Bill," he said, "tell me what's been happening since I left."
"Nothing. Nothing at all." said Bill.
"Aw c'mon, Bill. There had to be something that happened. Tell me, I don't care how piddling you think it is."
"Well...it's hard to think of anything. Except that your dog died."
"No! Old Blue? How'd that happen?"
"Can't say for sure. Vet thinks it's cuz he ate the burnt horse flesh."
"Burnt horse flesh! Where'd he get burnt horse flesh?"
"Well, when your barn burned down, none of the horses got out and he must have gotten in there and..."

"My barn burned? How'd that happen?"

"Can't say for sure. Fire marshal thinks the sparks from your house..."

"My house! My house burned?"

"Yep. Clear to the ground."

"My god, how'd that happen?"

"Can't say for sure. Marshall thinks one of the candles next to the coffin fell against the curtains and..."

"Coffin! What coffin?"

"Oh yeah, your mom died too."

"My mother died! How?"

"Can't say for sure. Doc thinks she died of a heart attack after your wife ran off with your hired hand."

The world loves smiles and laughter for the obvious reason that they are associated with good, warm feelings. On the other hand, tears, frowns, red faces and yelling are generally associated with anger, sadness and other negative emotions.

Do you smile more than you frown? _____

☐ SOURCES OF HUMOR

Caregiving is actually fertile ground for humor because of its affiliation with many of the conditions found on the dark side. Mark Twain recognized that when he said, *"The secret source of humor is not joy, but sorrow."*

Here are a half dozen sources of humor that can be found in caregiving—or life in general—that many humorists find to be the essence of humor. They include hostility, exaggeration, aggression, realism, tension and surprise. Interestingly, when taken together, they spell HEARTS, the depiction of love.

Hostility

Some caregivers develop feelings of hostility toward their care receiver, other family members or the health care agencies and professionals they must deal with. The most common expressions of hostility—and the jokes they sometimes generate—include the following:

1. **Family problems:** Henny Youngman, *"Take my wife...please!"*

2. **Sexual frustration:** Roger Dangerfield, *"If it weren't for pickpockets, I'd have no sex life at all."*

3. **Financial concerns:** John Barrymore, *"If it isn't the sheriff, it's the finance company; I've got more attachments than a vacuum cleaner."*

4. **Intrusion of authority into our private lives:** Barry Goldwater, *"A government that is big enough to give you all you want is big enough to take it all away."*

5. **Feelings of anxiety, apprehension and depression:** Woody Allen, *"More than any time in history, mankind faces a crossroads. One path leads to despair and utter hopelessness. The other, to total extinction. Let us pray we have the wisdom to choose correctly."*

6. **Lack of control of the technology in our environment:** Mark Russell, *"The scientific theory I like best is that the rings of Saturn are composed entirely of lost airline luggage."*

7.   Human characteristics or foibles which trigger our prejudices and taunts: David Frost, *"Television enables you to be entertained in your home by people you wouldn't have in your home."*

Exaggeration

Some jokes mix truth with an impossible exaggeration. Listeners know what they hear isn't true, but they enjoy the illusion. Stories of this type usually involve overstatement or understatement in the exaggeration. Phyllis Diller, *"There is so much crud in my oven there is only room to bake a single cupcake."*

Aggression

Many people feel like they don't stand a chance against lawyers, big government, the medical profession or insurance companies. They use jokes as substitutes for other, unacceptable means of aggression against people or things that frustrate them. Jewish parable, *"Two farmers each claimed to own a certain cow. While one pulled on its head and the other pulled on its tail, the cow was milked by a lawyer."*

Reality

Most good jokes state a bitter truth. The most universally accepted and easiest to understand jokes about reality are two-line jokes. The first line states a truth or element of reality; the second line changes the expected ending into a surprise. Two or more realistic but contrasting circumstances are united into one thought. Nikita Krushchev, *"Politicians are the same all over. They promise to build a bridge even when there's no river."*

Tension

A set-up establishes tension within a joke, then the punch line relieves it. Billy Connolly, *"Roses are red, violets are blue. I'm a schizophrenic and so am I."*

Surprise

Sometimes humor can startle you into laughing—like a curve ball that starts out straight, then bends to surprise the batter. P. G. Wodehouse, *"I don't know if you have ever leaped between the sheets, all ready for a spot of sleep, and received an unforeseen lizard up the left pajama leg. It's an experience which puts its stamp on a man."*

Looking for humor in caregiving is not simply a diversion, but rather an essential requirement for preserving your mental and physical health. Your success in discovering its magic depends on how good a sense of humor you have.

What is your major source of humor? _____

☐   **SENSE OF HUMOR**

Viktor Frankl, author of *Man's Search for Meaning* and Nazi prison camp survivor, had this to say: *"Humor is another of the soul's weapons in the fight for self-preservation. It is well known that humor, more than anything else in the human makeup, can afford an aloofness and an ability to rise above any situation, even if only for a few seconds."*

A sense of humor is both a cognitive and emotional process that is unique to every individual. It is spontaneous and often outlandish. It is a coping mechanism, a communication skill and a tool that promotes the psychological and physiological well-being of all who possess it.

A caregiver with a sense of humor sees the fun in everyday experiences. Those who have discovered the power of humor find that it performs a variety of functions. A sense of humor...

... eases tension.
... conveys goodwill.
... helps reassert control.
... makes care receivers feel better.
... serves as a useful teaching tool.
... influences thinking and attitudes.
... enhances and projects a favorable image.
... is a potent weapon that is hard-to-defend-against.
... reduces the embarrassment of mistakes and
     awkward moments.

Humor, in almost any form, can spontaneously relieve fear, anxiety, anger and depression. It can be used to enhance everyday living and quality of life. And it's bound to make your caregiving experience a better one—guaranteed.

Every individual has a unique sense of humor. Whatever you think is funny *is* funny. What other people will or will not laugh at is mainly determined by the way they were brought up and how they have adapted to their present station in life.

On a scale of 1 (low) to 10 (high), how would you rate your sense of humor?

___1 ___2 ___3 ___4 ___5 ___6 ___7 ___8 ___9 ___10

Think about your place on the scale. What will change—or maintain —your position? How will that make you a better caregiver?

☐   **HUMOR, HAPPINESS AND HEALTH**

"Laughter is a tranquilizer that has no side effects." - Arnold Glasow, American humorist.

More and more evidence is available showing that laughter and a good sense of humor can suppress the negative effect that the strain of caregiving has on emotions. If you have a strong sense of humor, you'll have fewer mood swings and greater resistance to caregiver stress. Your sense of humor will also temper the effect that stress has on your immune system and your susceptibility to certain infections. A sense of humor will lengthen your life, and your life will lengthen your sense of humor.

Two major things happen to you when you listen to a typical joke, comedy routine or funny story:

1.   Your muscle tension increases in anticipation of the climax, or punch line.
2.   Immediately following the punch line (assuming that you thought it was funny and started laughing), your chest, abdomen and facial muscles get a vigorous workout.

In convulsive laughter, where you really break up, you might roll on the floor, stomp your feet, clap your hands and otherwise wear yourself out. When the spasm of laughter subsides, your pulse rate drops below normal and your skeletal muscles become deeply relaxed. During the laughter response, your body is revitalized by what is sometimes called "internal massage". In his book, *Anatomy Of An Illness,* Norman Cousins called laughter a form of internal jogging.

Studies show that caregivers are more likely than non-caregivers to experience depression, anxiety and physical illness. The stress and isolation brought on by caregiving can lead to feelings of anger, resentment and grief. It can also place caregivers at greater risk for unhealthy behaviors such as overeating and substance abuse. Those who are recovering from addiction of any kind may find themselves at greater risk for relapse. A sense of humor is one of the best methods available for reducing those risks and ensuring a healthier life. Here's how it works.

☐   LAUGHTER AS A HEALER

"Laughing is the sensation of feeling good all over and showing it principally in one place." - Josh Billings, American humorist.

Laughter can cure almost anything a caregiver can encounter. It calms tempers, soothes jagged nerves, breaks the gloom of growing old and fills a room with sunshine and good cheer. It also aids digestion, keeps you alert and soothes arthritic pain. Laughter is the health of the soul. It's a potent antidote for most of the world's worst physical maladies and the best medicine there is for a long and happy life.

Laughter can even prevent some heart attacks by diffusing anger, which is often a precipitating factor that is especially felt by caregivers. And by alleviating depression—another caregiver problem—it may play a role in reducing the risk of cancer.

Many medical experts say that laughter is as good for those who are sick as it is for those who care for them and want to stay well. It's a fact that a good laugh is an excellent restorative as well as preventive medicine for anyone. You couldn't find a better elixir for your "caregiver's medicine chest." It's no wonder that caregivers who laugh, last.

How much laughter do you have in your medicine chest? _____

_____

☐   **LAUGHTER AS A STIMULATOR**

   "Laughing 100 times a day is the cardiovascular equivalent of 10 minutes of rowing." - Dr. William F. Fry, Stanford University.

   Laughter is a total body experience in which all the major systems participate. A good belly laugh exercises your heart as well as your circulatory and respiratory systems. Laugh out loud and your facial, shoulder and stomach muscles all get into the act.

   Laughter activates the creative center of your brain, stimulates your heart and endocrine system and gives your internal organs a strenuous workout. The "internal jogging" effect of laughter improves your digestion rate and reduces muscular tension. Even your arms and legs get a mini-workout during hearty laughter.

   In the stimulation stage of laughter, you experience an increase in heart rate, blood pressure and respiration. Your circulatory system increases oxygen exchange and speeds up transportation of blood substances to your body cells. Your diaphragm—the main muscle of respiration that's situated right behind your chest and abdomen— starts convulsing, and that exercises your lungs and gets you breathing faster. Your whole cardiovascular system benefits because of the increased oxygen in the blood stream.

How often do you get "fired up" by laughter? _____

_____

☐ LAUGHTER AS A TRANQUILIZER

"For fast-acting relief, try slowing down." - Lily Tomlin, American comedienne.

The period of stimulation caused by laughter is followed by a state of relaxation—similar to that experienced in aerobic exercise—in which your respiration, heart rate and blood pressure all go down. As your laughter subsides, your tension also decreases until it is substantially lower than it was before the humor hit you.

The decrease in tension can continue for up to 45 minutes. The greater the intensity of your laughter, the larger the decrease and the more long-lasting the effect. Isn't that a nice way to find respite from a stressful day of caregiving?

Laughter causes a loss of muscle tone, so muscle-related pains tend to vanish in the wake of a hearty guffaw. Laughter's ability to cause muscles to relax is of great value in the treatment of caregiver stress. It's hard to feel anxious and tense about caregiving when you feel as limp as a wet rag. The fact is, anxiety and laughter-induced muscle relaxation are wholly incompatible. It's like mixing water and oil.

The deep feeling of relaxation that comes as a byproduct of laughter also produces physiological changes in your body. The combination of frequent laughter and relaxation has been scientifically proven to give relief from insomnia, headaches, backaches, hypertension, hyperventilation and panic attacks. It even helps resolve sibling disputes, which seem to creep into caregiving situations from time to time.

As a psychological side benefit, laughter promotes feelings of inner peace, well-being and emotional balance. It serves as a coping strategy by reducing feelings of anxiety, tension and anger. Energy is conserved, your immune system is preserved and you are better prepared to handle stressful caregiving situations. That makes laughter one of the best tranquilizers available. And it's a heck of a lot cheaper than prescription drugs.

Laughter-induced relaxation has another benefit; it puts you in a better frame of mind to make use of the magical benefits of humor.

Many caregivers have found that the best opportunity they have for rest and relaxation is to be "on time" for a doctor's appointment.

What effect does laughter have on your state of mind? _____

_____

☐   ATTITUDE ADJUSTMENTS

"People that keep stiff upper lips find that it's damn hard to smile." - Judith Guest, American author.

Caregivers who have a hard time seeing and enjoying humor, or laughing at themselves and their problems, find difficulty in dealing with the stress of caregiving. In contrast, those with a solid sense of humor find it easier to handle their trials and tribulations.

It's a well-known fact that humor is the hole that lets the sawdust out of a stuffed shirt.

Happiness and positive attitudes don't come from doing what you like to do or getting what you want. *They come from liking what you have to do and wanting what you get.*

You can develop a positive approach toward caregiving and enhance your sense of humor by thinking funny thoughts and developing a happy, healthy attitude. Here are some attitude adjustments you can try whenever there's a break in your caregiving chores:

- Read funny books.
- Go to funny movies.
- Watch comedy shows on TV.
- Check out the comedy shelf at the video store.
- Let yourself laugh at things you think are funny.

You can find a wealth of helpful strategies for developing a positive approach to caregiving by reading *Positive Caregiver Attitudes*, another book in this caregiver survival series.

☐ DISARMING WITH HUMOR

"If you're going to tell people the truth, you'd better make them laugh. Otherwise they'll kill you. My method is to take the utmost trouble to find the right thing to say, and then say it with the utmost levity." - George Bernard Shaw, Irish playwright.

Humor has a way of relieving tension between people and of bringing about greater understanding between them. It's a great lubricant for caregivers and care receivers alike.

Caregivers with a sense of humor often use it to deal with difficult people—including their care receivers—or to get through difficult moments, especially those that are related to heavy-duty caregiving. They know they can solve caregiving problems a lot easier by saying things in jest rather than in frustration. Using their sense of humor in tense caregiving situations is the ultimate expression of being calm, cool and collected.

A sense of humor relieves anxiety, serves as an outlet for hostility and anger and helps you to take control and command of almost every caregiving experience. It's like *Aikido*, the Japanese martial art that uses the principles of nonresistance in order to win over an antagonist.

Instead of using aggressive moves, Aikido dismisses problem people by gently—but effectively—unbalancing their energy and momentum. In a battle of wits, humor is used like Aikido to turn aside verbal aggressors, including obnoxious co-workers, uncompromising bureaucrats, meddlesome bystanders and uncooperative care receivers.

You can see Aikido-like humor at work by watching politicians and nightclub comics handle hecklers. They're able to act with grace under pressure in tense, embarrassing, or "put-up or shut-up" moments. They control their interactions as effectively as former heavyweight champion Muhammed Ali, who could *"dance like a butterfly, sting like a bee."*

It's far better to be prepared and never use your Aikido responses than to be haunted by all the great, *"I should have saids,"* you should have said, and could have said.

Once while leaving a fancy Manhattan supper club, humorist Robert Benchley turned to the man in uniform at the door and said, *"Would you please get us a taxi?"*

The man stiffened pompously. *"I'm sorry,"* he replied icily, *"but I happen to be a Rear Admiral in the United States Navy."*

"All right, then," said Benchley, *"get us a battleship."*

That's Aikido.

Describe how you might have used Aikido (or tongue-foo) in some of your care giving experiences: _____

_____

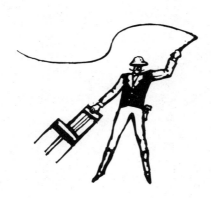

WHAT'S SO FUNNY?

☐ THE NEED FOR HUMOR

President Lincoln thought everyone needed a sense of humor, including himself. In the midst of a civil war that was tearing the nation apart, he said, *"With the fearful strain that is on me night and day, if I did not laugh, I should die."*

The common perception of humor is that it is fun, but it plays a much greater role than that. Humor helps you battle—with mental agility, rather than physical ability—the things that threaten you as a caregiver. It's probably the most effective way you have for getting through your darkest moments.

It's hard to find much to laugh about in caregiving, especially when your care receiver is difficult to care for. Disease, dementia, incontinence, disorientation and crippling injury are not fertile topics for stand-up comedians. But searching for humor in a caregiving environment is a lot better than focusing on elements that can torment you with anger, frustration or depression.

A situation that is extremely grave at the moment may bring a warm glow of happiness when it is recalled in less stressful times. Something that irritates you today may bring peals of laughter tomorrow. The right words spoken in a humorous vein can turn a difficult situation into a bond of understanding between you and your care receiver that will last for days.

A healthy sense of humor relieves anxiety and tension, serves as an outlet for hostility and anger, provides a healthy diversion, and lightens the heaviness of disability and illness. It also builds your self-confidence, enhances your physical health, increases your tolerance to stress and makes you a better companion.

A sense of humor will help you...

> ...outlast the intolerable.
> ...tolerate the unpleasant.
> ...overlook the unattractive.
> ...cope with the unexpected.
> ...smile through the unbearable.
> ...understand the unconventional.

There will always be times when the pain of caregiving overcomes you and your heart is filled with sadness. But those times will pass. They always do—when you let them. The difficult part is laughing at—and with—yourself and others without lessening the gravity of your task. In today's negative, bad news atmosphere, the challenge is even greater.

It is not demeaning to make light of serious information. Humor provides a useful tool for explaining anything, especially when what you're explaining is frightening, complicated, or very close to the heart. The Roman poet Horace recognized this when he said, *"A jest often decides matters of importance more effectively and happily than seriousness."*

Physiologically, there is little difference between laughter and sorrow. They're both a part of life, just like rain and sunshine are part of weather. Saying that there can be no laughter is like saying there can be no rain. Laughing and crying often go together. Sometimes you laugh so hard you cry. And when you cry a lot, you start to laugh. You're relieving tension whether you're laughing or crying. Of the two, laughter usually makes you feel better. It's just the ticket for a weary caregiver.

"If you can find humor in it, you can survive it." - Bill Cosby, American comedian.

□   WHO NEEDS IT?

It's estimated that 15 percent of American adults are providing special care for seriously ill and aging relatives and friends. That means there are about 7 million people like you in the United States alone who are struggling with the turbulent emotions and stressful responsibilities of caregiving.

Your needs are much the same. You long for the "three *Rs*" of caregiving: respite, recognition and resources.

- *Respite*–in the form of some quiet time by yourself.

- *Recognition*–in the form of emotional support from your care receiver and others for the hard work you're doing.

• **Resources**–in the form of information and financial assistance that will help you meet your needs and the needs of the person you're caring for.

You also need a lively sense of humor. Comedian Red Skelton recognizes this in the credo he lives by. *"Have a little laugh at life and look around you for happiness instead of sadness. Laughter has always brought me out of unhappy situations. Even in your darkest moment, you can usually find something to laugh about if you try hard enough."*

You're not alone in your need for humor, nor are you alone as a caregiver. Here's a capsule look at some of the people who are struggling with many of the same concerns that you are.

Caregivers in the United States average between 55 and 60 years old; 10 percent are over 75.

Care *receivers* range in age from the very young to the very old. Children and young adults who are disabled by injury or illness need just as much care as older people who have broken a hip or have to live with Alzheimer's disease.

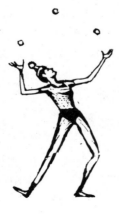

APPROXIMATELY 7,000,000 CAREGIVERS		
Characteristic	Percent	Number
Women	75 %	5,250,000
Men	25 %	1,750,000
Spouses	48 %	3,360,000
Adult children	34 %	2,380,000
Work outside home	25 %	1,750,000
44 years or younger	15 %	1,050,000
45-64	31 %	2,170,000
65 or older	55 %	3,850,000

You probably assist with daily living, performing such chores as grocery shopping, cooking meals and doing housework. You might also help with bathing, toileting, grooming and feeding or with financial routines like budgeting and check writing.

If you drive, you probably take your care receiver to doctor's visits and other destinations. You provide advice and support in decision making. You might even administer medications on a regular basis.

Not surprisingly, 75 percent of family caregivers in a recent study said if they quit taking care of their parents, it would reduce their parents' quality of life "a great deal" or even "unbearably".

> The average American woman spends 17 years of her life caring for children and 18 years helping aging parents. Do you wonder why so many women compare caregiving to laughing with a busted rib?

Do you as a caregiver, with your unique set of circumstances, have any special talents—or limitations—that affect your ability to give care?

My Response: _____

_____

☐   HUMOR AND YOUR CARE RECEIVER

"We cannot really love anybody with whom we never laugh." - Agnes Repplier, American essayist.

You may have difficulty in sharing humor with an impaired care receiver who is anxious, frustrated, combative, or standoffish. Don't let that change your course. Be persistent in creating an environment in which you can still maintain your sense of humor. This book will show you how to do that. It will also show you how the magic of humor can make your caregiving a much more positive experience.

The way you became a caregiver can influence your attitude toward caregiving. How *did* you become a caregiver?

_____ *I willingly chose to do it.*   _____ *I had no choice.*

If you chose to become a caregiver, you were probably motivated by love or guilt and based your decision on whether you had the time, energy, money or patience to do it.

If you had no choice, you probably found yourself suddenly and unexpectedly in a position that demands great personal sacrifice. You may be giving care because of a family commitment, limited financial resources, your proximity to the care receiver or the lack of anyone else to do the job. Or maybe you drew straws with your siblings and came out as the designated caregiver.

In any case, caregiving can disrupt your family life, put a strain on your resources and create emotional chaos. Some caregiving situations become disasters. But in most cases it's a positive experience that brings families together during a difficult time.

One of the hardest things you have to do as a caregiver is to *detach* yourself from your care receiver and take care of your own needs. Detachment means some or all of the following:

- being able to say *No!* (if only to yourself) without feeling guilty.

- making the most of what you have and not dwelling on what you've lost.

- thinking about the good years you've had and trying to make the most out of today.

- harnessing your anger and frustration so they don't cloud your thoughts about your care receiver.

A healthy sense of humor helps make it all happen. You cannot, however, inject humor into your caregiving at the expense of your care receiver. If you're both on the same humor track and can live and laugh *together* as caregiver and care receiver, then you're in luck. But what you may think is funny in one setting may seem harmful, insensitive and uncaring to someone else. If you're going in opposite directions, then you'll have to go it alone or find someone else with whom you can share your sense of humor. (We'll talk about "humor buddies" later.) The worst you can do is let your sense of humor die because your care receiver can't—or won't—laugh at anything.

Here are three categories that you should consider when you exercise your sense of humor.

1.   **For Your Funny Bone Only.** This category of humor includes funny things you do when you're by yourself to cheer yourself up. It's made up of things that only you would understand and appreciate. It could also include things you keep to yourself because you think they might upset your care receiver. It could be going through a scrapbook of cartoons or listening to oldtime radio tapes. For some of you, it might mean making funny faces in front of a mirror.

2.   **Testing the Waters.** There are some humorous things you can do with your care receiver that will help reduce the stress or tension that exists between you and let you both relax, even when your care receiver can't appreciate or understand your efforts.

     You may find a cartoon in the morning paper, for example, that really breaks you up. After patiently explaining it to your care receiver, you may find a broad smile or a vacant stare. You need to test your ideas from time to time until you know how much you can share. Just don't start out with a lampshade on your head.

3. **Shared Laughter**.   This category is made up of funny things you and your care receiver can enjoy together, at any time, that will help you both feel better. You might rent a video of a funny movie you both enjoyed. Or you could check out a book of old comedy routines from the library if you both enjoyed hearing them on the radio. You might also get out some old photo albums and recall some crazy episodes you may have experienced together. Old high school yearbooks are sure to generate a chuckle or two.

Do something in each of these three categories and you'll reduce the stress of caregiving, protect your mental and physical health and capture some of the magic of humor in caregiving. Share your humor with your care receiver and members of your support group. Spread lightheartedness around like homemade rhubarb jam so it sticks to everybody.

"You see things that are and say 'Why?' But I dream things that never were and say, 'Why not.'" - George Bernard Shaw, Irish playwright.

The next section introduces you to three major causes of caregiver problems. They are the ones that are most often encountered by caregivers who have lost their sense of humor—or never had much of one to start with.

THE COST OF SADNESS

☐ **FEAR OF FOOLISHNESS**

"The philosophies of one age have become the absurdities of the next, and the foolishness of yesterday has become the wisdom of tomorrow." - Sir William Osler, Canadian physician.

The fear of making a fool of yourself is deep-seated. Like many children, you were probably reprimanded back in elementary school for "acting silly." All it took to "shape you up" was a stern look from your teacher or a whack across your knuckles with a ruler. Now, a steely glare from your spouse, your boss, your pastor or the judge who acts on your speeding violation probably has the same effect.

When you were a kid, you wouldn't hesitate to lick jelly off a sharp knife. Now you almost have a heart attack when you see one of your children or grandchildren doing it.

You've developed a whole parcel of fears as you've aged, and many of them don't make sense. They only complicate your life and

make you miserable. Some fears are insignificant, the consequences wholly improbable. You might be like some people, for
example, who are afraid to tear the "DO NOT REMOVE UNDER
PENALTY OF LAW" label from their mattresses. Or you think you'll
get in serious trouble for having one extra item in the express
checkout line.

If the fear of foolishness has a grip on you, it's time to sort
through that fear and figure out what's causing it. Start by thinking
of the worst possible thing that could happen if you wore a Groucho
Marx nose and glasses while serving breakfast to your care receiver.
Or what kind of response do you suppose you'd get if you brought
balloons, whistles and funny hats to your caregiver support group?
Do you really think your doctor would throw you out of the
examination room if you showed up wearing "Elvis Is King!"
underwear at your next physical?

Write down, as clearly as you can, what you think would
happen to you if you really let your hair down—not just to your
shoulders, but all the way to your toes—and actually did something
silly.

     ☹   *My neighbors would call 911!*
     ☹   *I'd lose my subscription to* Library News!
     ☹   *My care receiver would refuse to talk to me!*

Prepare to accept each calamity as if the bogeyman was waiting
in the wings to pounce on you for doing it.

Once you've clearly stated your fear and prepared to be
skewered for doing it, write down as many ways as you can think of
for getting rid of it. Use your imagination and put down every
solution that comes to mind, no matter how crazy or unreasonable it
seems at first glance.

☺ *I'd invite my neighbors over to join me for a picnic in the backyard and ask the Good Humor driver to cater it.*

☺ *I'd share my copies of* Laughing Matters *with other members of my support group.*

☺ *I'd tell my care receiver to "Go fly a kite!" Then I'd go along and help get it up.*

Go through your list of solutions and choose the one you think is going to do the most to eliminate your fear of foolishness. Then hitch up your drawers, spit on your hands and tear that fear to shreds. Do it with the confidence of a kid running backwards up a theater aisle.

My greatest fear about using humor in caregiving is:_____

_____

☐ **ANGER**

"When angry, count four. When very angry, swear." - Mark Twain, American humorist.

Don't be afraid to express anger, because trying to hide it can cause more stress than letting it out. But be selective in how you express it. Instead of flying off the handle over every obstacle that gets in your way, use your anger to get around the obstacle and make improvements. Share your feelings with your support group. You'll find that many of the things you're mad about have probably bothered other caregivers. Just don't let anger consume you or corrupt your emotions.

One of the best ways to control anger is to observe the ridiculous nature of the situation that made you mad and then probe it for the humor it contains. If your care receiver throws his dinner against the kitchen wall, curb your anger and consider three courses of action:

1. Recognize that your care receiver's action was probably triggered by the nature of his illness or disability and was not an invitation for you to join him in a food fight.

2. If it is a food fight, try to outdo him by tossing your dinner with more flamboyance.

3. Ask him what he thinks about letting the mashed potatoes harden into a wall collage that the two of you could paint together.

Generally speaking, it's impossible for you to laugh and be angry at the same instant, because anger and laughter are mutually exclusive emotions. You have the power to choose which emotion is going to rule your behavior.

Whether you choose to laugh or get mad at life's aberrations probably won't matter much in the great scheme of things, except that laughter will fill your present moments with happiness and anger will waste them in misery. Just think, for every minute you're angry, you lose sixty seconds of peace of mind.

Here are some thoughts to keep in mind whenever your anger is about to overtake your sense of humor.

• The world needs more warm hearts and fewer hot heads.

- People who lose their heads are usually the last ones to notice.

- Have you ever noticed that a fire department never fights fire with fire?

- You are generally measured by the size of the things that make you mad.

- Just because you blow your top doesn't mean you have a dynamite personality.

- Angry caregivers are seldom reasonable; reasonable caregivers get angry, but they know how to control their feelings.

- Anger gets you into trouble because it makes your mouth move faster than your brain.

- Every time you give your care receiver a piece of your mind you make your head a little emptier.

Getting a handle on anger doesn't require a personality transplant, but you do have to become a better evaluator of yourself, your reactions and your priorities. You can't think clearly when you're angry, and if you can't think clearly, you can't be a very effective caregiver. American businessman Robert H. Ingersoll recognized the relationship between anger and thinking. *"Anger,"* he said, *"is a wind which blows out the lamp of the mind."*

How do you feel about the effects of anger? _____

_____

☐   STRESS AND TENSION

"Never do anything standing that you can do sitting, or anything sitting that you can do lying down." - Chinese proverb.

The stress and tension of caregiving stem from these three basic areas:

- Care receiver behavior and attitudes.
- Physical and emotional components of the illness or disability.
- Financial problems.

An imaginative sense of humor can help bring that stress and tension under control, regardless of where it comes from. Consider the three sources now and see if you can alleviate them with some of the magic of humor.

Care Receiver Behavior

People who live with illness or chronic pain often have bouts of depression. Others, such as people with Alzheimer's disease, experience serious personality changes. These care receivers are sometimes angry, unreasonable, unappreciative, or even unable to recognize their caregivers. Some may become violent or verbally abusive.

Disruptive behavior is often a consequence of a long-term disease or disability and not the result of deliberate action by a care receiver. Still, it's stressful for loving caregivers to maintain a sense of humor when their care is unrewarded or even thwarted.

Care receivers who have lost some of their mental faculties probably can't appreciate caregiver humor. It they can't understand it, they may misinterpret it. You can improve your caregiving experience by sharing as much of your humor as your care receiver can appreciate and doing your best to lighten their life. But you'll probably have to save the rib-tickling humor for yourself. At times it may be just the thing you need to keep from being swallowed up by your care receiver's stress-provoking behavior.

If you're just dealing with a grumpy care receiver, then fetch the heavy artillery. Call on your "humor buddies" for ammunition. Even if you're only partially successful in drawing out a laugh now and then from your care receiver, your efforts will still enrich your own humor capacity. You'll learn to use your sense of humor as a life preserver to keep from drowning under the stress of dealing with a cantankerous patient.

Physical and Emotional Concerns

Many caregivers have health problems of their own, but their problems often take a back seat to the demands of caregiving. They may, for example, find it easier to sink into the sofa and watch TV than to exercise or follow a balanced diet. Or they may skip regular physical exams because of difficulty in leaving their care receiver. Here's where a lighthearted approach to caregiving will save your day. If meals are a problem, keep leftovers in the freezer. Then once a week, or whenever a change is needed, use the leftovers for a picnic—summer *or* winter, inside *or* out. The change of pace will lighten your load *and* your heart.

Turn your checkup time into a self-renewal outing. Arrange for respite care through your church, support group, social service agency, or community resource center. (Check the list of resources in the back of this book for additional sources of help.) Then, while you have the time, check out a book on humor from your library, rent a comic video, or share some humor with friends.

Maintain contact with family and friends. Go to work on restoring your sense of humor through caregiver support groups. Establish a "humor squad" of caregivers like you who want to share their humor. Plan joint gatherings of caregivers and care receivers where everyone can lighten up.

Expand your resources and seek help from social service agencies and organizations. They're set up to help locate support groups and assist caregivers with ideas and strategies.

> Surveys have found that almost 25 percent of all primary caregivers have no one with whom they can discuss their physical, emotional or financial problems. Slightly less than half of the caregivers said their immediate families had no idea how much care they were giving. Considering the lack of people contact, it's not surprising that the rate of depression among caregivers is double that among non-caregivers of equivalent age, health and social status.

Financial and Legal Problems

Like many other caregivers, you may be employed outside your home. Or you may have had to give up your job or at least cut back on work hours to provide adequate care. Your loss of income is probably compounded by the fact that you are now spending up to 10 percent of your monthly income on expenses for a dependent care receiver. That creates a lot of stress, but not so much that it can't generate some humor.

You've probably heard many people talk about their financial problems. Get them in a group and they begin a game of one-upmanship. *"You think you have it tough, let me tell you how hard it is for us."* Pretty soon their conversations are lightened up with a touch of humor.

If there's nothing in your immediate future that's going to make your financial picture better, then you might be able to get rid of or eliminate some of your stress by injecting a bit of humor. All it needs is a little imagination and exaggeration.

"We have it so tough I can't even buy my kid a yo-yo for Christmas. All I can afford is a yo."

"We've got it so tough that now we only have two meal choices—take it or leave it."

Take positive steps to reduce your stress and tension by looking at the lighter side of caregiver behavior, physical and emotional concerns, and financial and legal problems.

Which of the above three sources causes you the most stress and tension and why do you think that's the case? _____

_____

☐ ONWARD AND UPWARD

"Life is too important to be taken seriously."- Oscar Wilde, Anglo-Irish playwright, novelist.

There is nothing funny about sickness or disability. And yet, some of the greatest comic routines that have ever been done have been developed around situations in which someone is sick or disabled. Lucille Ball, Red Skelton, Phyllis Diller, Laurel and Hardy, the Marx brothers and countless others have made us laugh at contrived dilemmas that are not unlike those you might find in caregiving.

The tension-filled situations that comedians create can be so awful that laughter is the only way to escape them. You probably can't escape from caregiving, but you can use humor as a release of tension, an escape from stress, or a defense against depression. A well-tuned sense of humor can restore the hope and energy you need to survive the realities of long-term illness or disability.

You don't have to look far to find the magic of humor in caregiving. Your daily life is rich with humor; it's all around you. It's just harder to find on some days than others. The trick is to clearly understand the many—and often confusing—elements of caregiving, then mine them for the humorous gems they contain. Sometimes it will test your creative abilities and at other times, the funny aspect of a caregiving situation will smack you right in the face like a custard pie.

HOW TO APPLY THE MAGIC

■ THE BASICS

"Comedy is simply a funny way of being serious." - Peter Ustinov, English actor.

You need a sense of humor for two main reasons:

a) to survive the rigors of caregiving.
b) to maintain your general mental and physical well-being.

It's much easier to enrich your sense of humor if your care receiver and others are in harmony with your efforts. By including friends and family, you have a ready audience for your efforts at mirth. Their positive response will give you the encouragement you need to add more humor to your life.

You could, of course, develop a good sense of humor without including your care receiver or anyone else. If you did that, you'd still make life a little bit better for yourself. But you'd be battling through the stress of caregiving alone without the magic that could make your efforts so much easier.

In the sections that follow, you'll find several strategies for strengthening your sense of humor and increasing your quota of giggles. Study them carefully and use those that work best for you. If you can think of some that are better than the ones presented, then by all means write them down and use them whenever possible.

■   **KNOW YOURSELF**

The first thing you should do is assess your humor capacity. Your answers to the following questions will tell you how much of a factor humor is—or has been—in your caregiving.

1.   On a scale of 1 (*low*) to 10 (*high*), what value do you place on a sense of humor? _____

2.   How often (*never–rarely–sometimes–often*) do you find yourself enjoying some humorous event that's related to caregiving?_____

3.   Have you been using humor *more, less, or the same* since you became a caregiver?_____

4.   Put a check mark (✔) in the space before each of the following activities that make you laugh:

_____   *cartoons*
_____   *joke books*

_____ *joke telling*
_____ *comedy cassettes*
_____ *comedy films or videos*
_____ *being around a funny person*
_____ *things my care receiver says and does*
_____ *other (please describe)* _____

_____

5. Is caregiving easier when your care receiver shows a sense of humor?

    _____ *Yes*   _____ *No*   _____ *Sometimes*

6. Is caregiving easier when other people (*family, friends, support group*) show a sense of humor?

    _____ *Yes*   _____ *No*   _____ *Sometimes*

7. How often (*never–rarely–sometimes–often*) does your sense of humor make you feel better or help you cope with the stress of caregiving? _____

8. Do you enjoy telling jokes or humorous stories to your care receiver? _____ To others (*family, friends, support group*)?

    _____

9. When do you find humor and laughter to be absolutely out of place? _____

    _____

10. Do you consider a sense of humor to be an essential part of caregiving? _____ Why (or why not)? _____

    _____

There are no right or wrong answers to the preceding questions. They're listed only as a way for you to measure your humor capacity and gain more insight into the relationship between humor and caregiving.

Your humor capacity will tell you a lot about your sense of humor, as well as your anxieties, concerns, emotional state and coping style. In order to experience more fully the magic of humor in caregiving, you need to check your humor capacity regularly and fill it whenever it gets low. A good time to start is right now.

My Strategy: _____

_____

■   KNOW YOUR CARE RECEIVER

"The audiences were really tough—they used to tie their tomatoes on the end of a yo-yo so they could hit you twice." - Bob Hope, American comedian.

Get to know as much as you can about your care receiver's sense of humor to see how easy it will be to develop your own. See if he or she reacts to the same kinds of humor that you do. Measure their humor capacity the same as you do your own. Find out if they share your likes and dislikes of jokes, comedians and humorous parodies. If they do, then you've got a wonderful humor partner and a great potential for some lighthearted caregiving.

Be sure you know if your care receiver is **ha ha**-ing or hurting when you try to share your mirth. Read the statements below and check (✔) those that you believe to be true of your care receiver. Your answers will give you a good idea of how much humor your care receiver can tolerate.

MY CARE RECEIVER'S SENSE OF HUMOR	✔ TRUE
Humor has always been a part of my care receiver's lifestyle.	
My care receiver's sense of humor is sincere and deep seated.	
My care receiver can communicate more effectively by using humor.	
A sense of humor has helped maintain my care receiver's physical well-being.	
My care receiver has effectively used humor in coping with illness and disability.	
A sense of humor helps my care receiver maintain a positive outlook for the future.	

If you checked *true* for 3 or more items, then chances are good that your care receiver would be receptive to a little bit of humor. All you need to do now is find out what things you can share.

Here are some questions you might ask yourself:

- Does my care receiver get a bigger kick out of comedy films or movies as opposed to reading or listening to jokes, cartoons, or funny stories? _____

- What kind of humor does my care receiver like best (puns, satire, wordplay, slapstick, burlesque, ethnic humor, limericks)? _____

- What things does my care receiver think are not funny?

    _____

Make a list right now of some of the things that have made you *and* your care receiver laugh in the past and would probably stir up some chuckles again.

☺ _____

☺ _____

☺ _____

☺ _____

☺ _____

☺ _____

See if there is a consistent pattern in the humorous things you and your care receiver share. If there is, then follow that pattern whenever you can to strengthen your own sense of humor and build a stronger "humor bond" between the two of you.

Try new sources of humor, but do so cautiously. If it's something that gives you belly laughs and your care receiver belly aches, then save it for a time when you can enjoy it by yourself.

Learn to appreciate and enjoy humor *together* and you will discover a time-proven method for coping with caregiver stress.

My Strategy: _____

_____

■ LAUGH AT YOURSELF

"He is not laughed at, that laughs at himself first." - Thomas Fuller, English clergyman and author.

Your ability to laugh at yourself is the most important ingredient in your recipe for enriching your sense of humor. It will help you grapple with all the oddball social, psychological and physiological events and processes that you run into every day as a caregiver. It will shape your caregiving like nothing else.

Laugh at yourself, not with ridicule, but with objectivity and acceptance of who and what you really are: a person who can make mistakes and not be afraid to admit it. Do it without reservation and your sense of humor will stay at full capacity.

> The young woman approached the employment
> interview with apprehension, knowing that a first
> impression could make or break her chances. But when
> she opened the door and walked toward the committee,
> her shoe caught on the carpet and she fell flat on her face.
> Without missing a beat, she got to her feet, smiled, and
> said, *"I always try to fall in with the right crowd."* She got
> the job.

Defuse criticism with humorous comebacks and silly squelches. Learn to take critical comments in a humorous light even if they are meant to embarrass you. If you take yourself too seriously, you can rest assured that no one else will.

Develop an accurate perception of yourself as you and others see you. Identify and accept those unique characteristics that complement your sense of humor. Recognize physical characteristics that you would like to change but can't (big ears, bald head) as well as traits that you may not wish to change (lightheartedness, a lover of animals).

Focus on characteristics that may be considered unusual, different, or mischievous. Emphasize your age, shape, color or ethnic diversity. If you've ever enjoyed the humor of Garrison Keillor on *The Prairie Home Companion,* you know how the Danes, Finns, Swedes and Norwegians in the Midwest have been poking fun at each other for years.

Look yourself over with a humorous eye. Acknowledge any shortcomings you might have in cooking, singing, or walking and chewing gum at the same time. Make a list of some of your biggest bonehead blunders and think about sharing them with others.

Erma Bombeck and Phyllis Diller have shared their unsophisticated housekeeping habits with audiences for years and have made a very good living doing it.

There are bound to be occasions in family, social, or business gatherings when one of your experiences will bring peals of laughter. Rely on the words of the English poet, George Gascoigne, *"An error gracefully acknowledged is a victory won. To make mistakes is human; to stumble is commonplace; to be able to laugh at yourself is maturity."*

You'll make more friends if you're able to laugh at yourself, because you'll be seen by others as being more attractive, warmer, confident and accepting. When you laugh at yourself, your care receiver and others will assume that you're not going to judge them more harshly than you judge yourself. They'll feel more at ease and not worry as much about making mistakes.

Take your caregiving responsibilities seriously, but take yourself lightly. You'll be a lot happier and life's anxieties and burdens will seem much lighter.

My Strategy: _____

_____

■   **LIGHTEN UP**

Sebastian Chamfort, the French satirist, said, *"The most utterly lost of all days is one in which you have not once laughed."* He obviously knew the value of laughter in relieving caregiver stress.

It's a common misconception that care receivers who are disabled because of illness or injury are always sad and have a despairing attitude. And as a caregiver, you're supposed to wear a long face too. That's just not so. A sense of humor is not a special characteristic that's reserved for the hale and hearty or for those who never deal with people who need care. It's a necessary component of everybody's personality. And with practice and dedication, it can be cultivated like any good habit.

If you can find something to laugh at, no matter how serious your situation is, you'll see caregiving in a new and refreshing way. That doesn't mean you're being disrespectful of your care receiver or the condition that brings you together. Nor does it mean that you have to find humor in everything. It just means you've tried to lighten the impact of one of life's misfortunes and tried to make your situation more enjoyable.

When a "disaster" occurs, label it as such, then flip it over and change it into something funny. If your care receiver spills a glass of milk, think of a cow that has sprung a leak. If you forget to pay the utility bill, think of being absconded by martians. A funny focus can get you out of a problem and into a solution before you know it.

Humor is also a great teacher. If you seek to find humor in an unhappy or embarrassing experience from your past, you'll probably uncover a lot of other emotions that were prominent at the time. Anger and frustration were probably the first to appear, with depression close behind.

Try it now. Focus on something you did that—after you think about it—was a little goofy, and see what you can learn about yourself. If you don't think you did anything funny, ask your friends. They might be able to come up with something, like the time you locked yourself out of your house, or the time you called 911 because you thought the meter-reader was a burglar.

Think of the goofiest thing you've done as a caregiver in the recent past. Describe it as you remember it or as others have described it to you. Then tell what you learned from it, now that the wounds have healed.

☆   This is the goofiest thing I've ever done as a caregiver: _____

_____

☆   This is how I felt when I did it: _____

_____

☆   This is what I learned from the experience: _____

_____

You may have thought what you did was traumatic when you did it, but when one of your favorite comics—like Lucille Ball or Robin Williams—did something similar, you probably thought it was hilarious.

Laughter is therapeutic. Every time you laugh, it makes you feel good, and feeling good improves your quality of life and increases your will to live. Psychologist William James said, *"We don't laugh because we're happy—we're happy because we laugh."* So whenever you have a chance to grin, giggle, smile and laugh at yourself, grab it. You might be surprised at the results.

Make up your mind to lighten up whenever your burden gets you down. You'll have fewer problems to worry about, and you will find greater pleasure in the person you care for. Avoid anger and dis-satisfaction, otherwise your work will drag on, you'll make mistakes and people will go out of their way to avoid you.

Develop a happy, healthy attitude by thinking positive thoughts and doing positive things. Look for expressions of joy and happiness in your environment. Be selective in the books you read and in the TV, movies, or videos you watch. Look for things that will reinforce your sense of humor, and allow yourself the pleasure of laughing at things you think are funny.

My Strategy: _____

_____

■   **SMILE**

"A smile is a curve that sets everything straight." - Phyllis Diller, American comedienne.

A lighthearted approach to living is usually demonstrated through facial expressions, which can convey all kinds of emotions to others. When you're smiling, your care receiver is going to feel much better about your relationship than if you were frowning all the time.

An unexpected smile is like a flash of lightning in the middle of a storm. It breaks through the clouds of gloom and lights up the world around you. A smile may only last a moment, but its effect can last a lifetime.

One of the laws of nature says that emotions cannot exist independently from their respective physical expressions. It's difficult, for example, to wear a sincere smile and feel sad at the same time.

It works the other way too. It's hard to wear an angry frown when you're deliriously happy. Your facial expressions cause changes in your involuntary nervous system, and that reinforces an appropriate emotion. That means you can alter your mood with a grin or a frown. So if you want to feel better, and make other people feel better too, put on a smile and watch what happens.

If you make a habit of smiling, people will think you're crazy and wonder what you're up to. Try smiling your way through the checkout line the next time you're at the market. Before long everybody else will get caught up in your enthusiasm for life and they'll be smiling too. Smiles and laughter are like perfume. You can't spray them on others without getting a little on yourself.

My Strategy: _____

_____

■ BUILD YOUR SELF-ESTEEM

"Be a friend to yourself, and others will be so too." - Thomas Fuller, English clergyman and author.

Your self-esteem reflects the way you feel and think about yourself. It's your belief in what you can and cannot do and is measured by the way you act. It is the keystone that holds your sense of humor in place.

Having high self-esteem means acting in a positive and optimistic manner, accepting your overall strengths and weaknesses and taking responsibility for your feelings, desires, thoughts, abilities and interests. Strengthen your self-esteem and you will strengthen your sense of humor. Strengthen your sense of humor and you will gain greater control of your entire life.

The way you feel about yourself and the world you live in is also going to determine how good a caregiver you're going to be. If you're happy and give your sense of humor a good workout, the years will be full of promise. If you go through life being angry, frustrated, or depressed, you'll be as miserable as an underwear salesman in a nudist camp.

It's generally agreed by professionals and nonprofessionals alike that people who feel good about themselves and have high self-esteem make better caregivers. If, on the other hand, you put a small value on your ability as a caregiver, you can rest assured that no one else will raise your price.

If you're like most caregivers, you like people who make you laugh. If you make people laugh, chances are they will like you just as well. And when other people like you, you get along with them much better. Finding the same thing funny as another person is not only a prerequisite to a real friendship, but often the first step in its formation.

Humor also helps create and enhance your personal image. Instead of coming across like a confused, red-faced nincompoop whenever you make an embarrassing mistake or find yourself in an awkward situation, respond with a lighthearted comment. The right response can sometimes make for an instant recovery.

> The caregiver who accidentally knocked her neighbor's glasses in the toilet, leaned down and asked,
> *"Now, can you folks see better down there?"*

The desire to improve your self-esteem must come from within, no one else can give it to you. Once you have the desire, and maintain it, it will motivate you more than any other force.

Present yourself as a confident caregiver. Maintain a healthy mind and body. Know your strengths and play up your strong features. Strive to maintain a positive connection between your self-image and your sense of humor. If you don't control the way you look at life, someone else will direct your vision.

Identify with people who share your outlook on life. Discover the beliefs and strategies that they've used to develop their self-esteem, and rework them for your own use. Good role models can save you months, even years, of trial and error. Henry Ford once said, *"Your best friend is whoever brings out the best in you."* Follow Ford's advice and associate with people from whom you can draw guidance and inspiration. A caregiver support group is an excellent place to start making contacts.

Focus on the things you're able to achieve with a lighthearted approach. Don't play down the seriousness of caregiving, just remember the power that lies in the magic of humor. Recall the effect it has on your physical and mental well-being. Know the effect it has on your care receiver and other people with whom you come in contact.

My Strategy: _____

■ LOOK FOR HUMOR EVERYWHERE

Remember the words of Dr. Seuss, *"From there to here, from here to there, funny things are everywhere."*

The magic of humor can be found in caregiving only after you fully understand your care receiver's condition and your ability to cope with it. Learn about symptoms, prognosis, rehabilitation and the likelihood of improvement or the probability of decline. Know when to get in touch with doctors and other health professionals. And know what to expect from your care receiver and others when you try to add a touch of humor to your caregiving.

Look for the funny or flip side of every aspect of caregiving no matter how painful it may be. Begin each week with an anecdote or funny joke that's related to some caregiving problem that will have to be tackled before the week is through. Do it daily if time and circumstances permit.

Take a few minutes to look for jokes, puns, satire, or even a little bit of old-fashioned corn that's tasteful, reflects your personality and won't offend your care receiver—or anyone else with whom you share your humor.

Scan your morning paper for humorous items. Admittedly there's not much to laugh about in today's news, but you can always find a hilarious cartoon in the comics section or on the editorial page. Political cartoons usually bust up half the readers and offend the other half. You've got a better than average sense of humor if you can laugh at most of them.

It's rare, but some radio personalities still prefer lighthearted humor to a call-in format. Spin your dial and see if you can find someone you like. Look for humorous stories in newsletters or magazines that come to your door. When you find something that tickles your funny bone and can be used in caregiving, cut it out and paste it in a scrapbook or write it down in a journal. (Use a *Dr. Seuss Journal* as explained in the next section.)

Call a ***humor buddy***—someone in your caregiver support group, or a friend, neighbor or relative that you can turn to on a regular basis. Your list of humor buddies should include people who are most likely to say and do funny things, or are the most likely to share humorous thoughts that they know you would appreciate. Borrow bits of humor from them whenever you can. Work with them to develop a humorous approach to current caregiving problems.

Get in the habit of asking yourself probing questions, like these:

"What's so amusing about what just happened or what I just saw or read?"

"Will this be humorous when I tell it later?"

"Wouldn't it be funny if..............................?"
  (let your mind wander).

Feel good about your ability to find humor in disheartenment. It will help keep you socially active and physically and mentally healthy. It will give you respite from stress and provide a warm and enjoyable environment for both you and your care receiver.

"If something wonderful happens to you—remember that! Those are the precious moments that carry you through the bad times. Nobody goes through life laughing all the time. If you can think of the nice things— even the little things—then you've got the day made." – Sid Caesar, American comedian.

My Strategy: _____

_____

■   **KEEP A DR. SEUSS JOURNAL**

Once you find useful tidbits of humor, you should have a good place to keep them. It's easy and fun when you have a *Dr. Seuss Journal.*

A *Dr. Seuss Journal* is a day-to-day accounting of ideas, events, reflections and experiences that stimulate your sense of humor and ease the burden of caregiving. Your notes, jokes and anecdotes don't have to be lengthy or time-consuming, just a line or two that will give you some insight into your feelings.

Write down the happy and sad things that happen to you in a day and tell how you respond to them. See if you can find a humorous side to the sad ones, and get another giggle out of the funny things that made you laugh.

Consult your *Dr. Seuss Journal* often. Over time, it will tell you what you've done in the past, show where you are in the present and help you chart a course for the future. It will remind you of what you once thought was funny and what now doesn't seem so sad after it's been laid to rest. Your history of emotional responses will tell you how you reacted to the experiences of daily living as well as a variety of caregiving obstacles and opportunities.

Your *Dr. Seuss Journal* will also provide a soothing, relaxing way to get in touch with your thoughts and feelings. It will allow you to reflect on positive as well as negative feelings that you might not want to express to others, including your care receiver. Expressing your feelings in the haven of your own written record will reduce stress, promote good mental and physical health and encourage you to get to know yourself a little better.

You can list events the way you would in a diary, but you should also include concerns, opinions and reflections about the meaning of your actions. If you have a problem figuring out what you want to say, just ask yourself some simple questions, like the following:

"How did I feel when...................happened?"

"Why did I feel that way?"

"How can I recapture (or avoid) that feeling?"

It's amazing how quickly the most seemingly unforgettable ideas vanish when you don't write them down. So keep pen and paper or a small tape recorder with you at all times. Remember that, *"the faintest ink is better than the best memory."*

Don't despair if you find it hard to write things down. American author Gene Fowler felt the same way when he said, *"Writing is easy; all you do is sit staring at a blank sheet of paper until the drops of blood form on your forehead."*

My Strategy: _____

_____

■ BUILD A HUMORTORIUM

Pursue the magic of humor by letting the little child in you come out to play. Start by establishing what humorist Jeanne Robertson calls a "humortorium." It's a place in which you keep funny books, tapes, cartoons, videos and other such mirth makers as balloons, clown noses or bottles of bubble soap. It's a good place to keep your *Dr. Seuss Journal.*

Your humortorium can take up an entire room or be squeezed into a broom closet. Decorate it to your heart's content to remind yourself, your care receiver and visitors that it's the place to go to take a "humor break."

Search for items to put in your humortorium whenever you have a chance. Read the advice columns in your local newspaper. Ask questions and take notes at your caregiver support group sessions. Send for materials from organizations that specialize in helping caregivers find the humor in living and caregiving. (The Humor Project, Inc., 110 Spring Street, Saratoga Springs, New York, 12866 is an excellent place to start.)

Be playful, even childlike, whenever possible in an environment (active caregiving) that is often thought to be extremely serious. Lighten up a stressful caregiving atmosphere by cutting loose from your usual mode of thinking. Use the material in your humortorium to find a new and creative way of providing care. If done well, you'll improve your sense of humor, reduce your stress and best of all, you'll make life better for your care receiver.

My Strategy: _____

_____

■ CREATE YOUR OWN HUMOR

For some, creating humor is easier said than done. But by using the following strategies, you may have a lot fewer problems than you anticipate. Try applying each of these blockbusting verbs to your task and see if you can't generate a little magic on your own. Some off-the-wall examples are provided for each category.

Substitute: What can you substitute as an expression of your feelings about caregiving instead of anger or frustration? Are there other characteristics that you can put in place that will reduce stress and tension for you and your care receiver? What words can you use other than pain, dementia, incontinence or depression that will lighten your load? Is there another tone of voice you can use in addressing your problems?

Examples: Paint funny faces on balloons and complain to them instead of to your care receiver or others. Tie the balloons to the backs of chairs and invite them for a conversation-filled meal.

Combine: How can you blend tasks, ideas and emotions into a collage of caregiving humor? Is there an assortment of jokes, songs, cartoons, limericks, or audio and video tapes that will improve your sense of humor and bring pleasure to your care receiver?

Examples: Start meals with a lighthearted song, naps with a funny story, baths with a shower of multicolored bubbles and trips to the doctor with a stop for ice cream cones.

Rearrange: Can you interchange the elements of caregiving to allow time for the development of humor? Can you change the pace of caregiving by rearranging habitual patterns of behavior?

Examples: Rearrange visits by social workers and home health aides. Have them come at varying times if possible. Start each day earlier, take short catnaps when you can, stay up a little later at night for a bit of reading or meditation.

Reverse: How can you change your caregiving situation from negative and sad to positive and pleasant? What is opposite of what you fear? Can you find humor by looking at your problems backwards or upside down? Can you reverse your role, change positions, turn the tables, or turn the other cheek?

Examples: *Turn a "**consequences of**..." list into a "**wish for**..." list. Match your list of aggravations with an equal number of blessings.*

Adapt: Have you had to face problems like this before? What solution did you think of then? What can you copy? Who can you imitate?

Examples: *Consult photo albums, old diaries, military history, school or work experiences, or the memory of friends and relatives to get a sense of what you did in the past.*

Modify: Can you give your caregiving a new twist by changing colors, sounds, smells, tastes, or shapes? Are there other changes in what you are doing now that will lighten your life and make you and your care receiver happier?

Examples: *Use paint, music, potpourri, fresh baked goods or cuddly teddy bears to stimulate your senses and improve your caregiving environment.*

Magnify: What can you add to make your situation better? How can you get more time? What can you do with greater frequency? Can you make something stronger, higher, or longer? Can you duplicate, multiply, or exaggerate something?

Examples: *Get a BIG kitchen clock so you're more conscious of seconds, minutes and hours. Then try to manage your time like money.*

Minimize: What can you subtract to make your problems smaller, shorter, or lighter? Can some of your caregiving responsibilities be condensed, omitted, streamlined, split up or understated?

Examples: *Have a friend or support group member watch how you do things, and see what time-wasting chores can be eliminated.*

These eight verbs form the acronym **SCRAM**. It's shorthand for **S**ubstitute, **C**ombine, **R**earrange, **R**everse, **A**dapt and **M**odify, **M**agnify, **M**inimize. SCRAM was described in a slightly different context in *Creative Caregiving,* another book in the *Caregiver Survival Series.* Think SCRAM whenever you need to create more humor and less stress in your caregiving situation.

"In creating, the only hard thing's to begin. The grass blade's no easier to make than an oak." - James Russell Lowell, American poet, critic, editor and diplomat.

My Strategy: _____

_____

■ PRACTICE MENTAL IMAGERY

"You can't depend on your judgment when your imagination is out of focus." - Mark Twain, American humorist.

Use mental imagery to replace sad thoughts with happy thoughts. Picture a smile ☺ on the face of the grouch behind the pharmacy counter. Open your memory bank and recall happy times and humorous events that made you laugh. Vaporize bad moods with your martian ray gun and replace them with nonsensical parodies.

Use positive imaging to create a picture in your mind's eye of the successful caregiver you want to be. See yourself as stronger, more relaxed, more confident and better able to handle stress. Hold the picture in your thoughts until your focus is clear.

The image you see will give you a realistic idea of what you need to do to restore your self-esteem and introduce the magic of humor into caregiving. Bring that image into view whenever you run into a seemingly impossible problem or unexpected obstacle. Imagine, for example, the progress you could make if you used mental imagery to create your humortorium and all it should contain.

Use the imagery of fantasy and daydreams to increase your capacity for humor and create feelings of well-being and happiness. Zero in on a single positive detail of caregiving, like the smile that will be on the face of your care receiver when you've added some humor to both of your lives.

Let your focus spread until you see your entire caregiving role in a positive way. Entertain dreams of unfounded optimism and exaggerated feelings of control. Become the ***Jolly Green Giant*** of caregiving.

Practice mental imagery by creating other visions in which you can see things move. Picture a flower growing from seed, water flowing through a creek, horses running in the wind, clowns getting out of a tiny car, snow decorating a pine tree or anything else that tickles your fancy. These illusions will serve as "warm up" exercises for creating visual solutions for a variety of caregiving problems.

Mental imagery is healthy and easy to do and can provide you with a ready source of fun and encouragement. You won't always accomplish everything you visualize, but you'll do much better than if you never imagined anything at all. Practice it whenever you can.

My Strategy: _____

_____

■ WORK AT IT

"If you're going to take Vienna—take Vienna!" - Napoleon Bonaparte, Emperor of France.

Learn something new about the magic of humor every chance you get. It can be as simple as learning the proper way to tell a joke, or as complex as learning about the therapeutic benefits of humor. Read humorists like Erma Bombeck, Art Buchwald, Mark Twain, Garrison Keillor, or any of a host of others.

Think creatively in a "what if" situation. Pick an interesting story out of your daily newspaper, and think how it would turn out *"if "* it had a hilarious twist to it. What *if* your favorite politician were to make a major blooper on the floor of Congress? What *if* your favorite football player were to score a touchdown for the other team? What *if* Air Force One landed the President in the wrong city?

Try the same approach on the routine tasks you do as a caregiver. Write down your *"what if"* endings and see if there is a speck of humor among them. If there is, take it and make it work for you.

ROUTINE TASKS	WHAT IF...
Feeding	The Hotel Ritz offered to cater all your meals for a year.
Laundry	Your washing machine refused to give back matched pairs of socks.
Housework	Your house was picked for next week's "Parade of Homes" tour.
Check writing	The bank mistakenly credited your account for $1,000,000.00.
Grocery shopping	You found a coupon in the cereal box for a Caribbean cruise.

If you have the time to watch TV, select special programs that will strengthen your sense of humor. Avoid those that make you sad. Watch comedy specials on cable or public television. Follow up the programs with a trip to the library, then check out books, videos or cassette tapes that you and your care receiver can both enjoy.

Whenever time permits, write jokes, poems, essays, short stories, or funny letters to friends and relatives. Write about the funny episodes in your family history. Create a funny story with you and your care receiver as major characters. Keep whatever you write in your *Dr. Seuss Journal.* Save the good stuff, improve what you can and toss the rest.

Rehearse new jokes and commit them to memory before you tell them to your care receiver or humor buddies. Memorize rhymes, riddles and poems that will make you laugh, and call them up whenever you need a "humor fix." If you have trouble remembering them, then check out a memory improvement book from your local library.

My Strategy: _____

_____

■ **CHANGE THE ATMOSPHERE**

"The more things change, the more they remain the same."
- Alphonse Karr, French journalist and novelist.

Establish a caregiving environment where a lighthearted approach is allowed and encouraged. Feel free to express your sense of humor and don't be afraid of making a fool of yourself. Your approach to caregiving should not be based on other people's criteria of what's proper and what's not.

Allow yourself to make an occasional mistake without feeling embarrassed. Analyze your goof-ups to determine their source. Learn from them, then let them go. Develop new strategies that will protect your self-esteem and give you the confidence it takes to try again.

Establish a safe, open and permissive environment in which responsibilities and commitments are combined with the magic of humor. Build an atmosphere in which you and your care receiver can feel comfortable sharing joys and laughter without the "fear of foolishness." Avoid "group-think" where you become more interested in getting the approval of others than trying to come up with lighthearted solutions to the problems at hand. If your critics persist, invite them into your humortorium for a little brain-cleansing.

My Strategy: _____

_____

■ CONNECT WITH HUMOR

"Friendships improve happiness and abate misery by doubling our joy and dividing our grief." - Joseph Addison, English essayist.

Laughter is a social event. You don't laugh when you tickle yourself, you laugh when someone else tickles you.

Reinforce your sense of humor by sharing it with as many people as you can. Begin at home by helping your spouse, parents, children or care receiver add more humor and laughter to their lives. Then work on your neighbors, friends or co-workers. You may not be successful with everyone, but the process is guaranteed to make you a happier person.

Seek the stimulation of someone older than you who has maintained a rich sense of humor. Seek the enthusiasm and naivete of someone younger who might have a whole different perspective on what's funny and what's not. Both can provide stimulation, direction, guidance and reflection, all of which are essential ingredients for creating humor.

Ask this question of the people you share with, *"What's the funniest thing that happened to you today?"*

Ask them to expand on the funny things they've seen or heard. If it's something you think is funny, then ask permission to share their experience with others. Let them know that you're a listener of good humor—not humor that's in bad taste or puts people down. If they know you're genuinely interested, they will search you out when they have another funny story to tell. Your *humor connections* will provide you with a rich source of material as well as lasting friendships. Once you've got people laughing with you, you've got them as friends.

Work with *humor buddies,* including—if possible—your care receiver. Seek out people like you who understand the magic of humor and the importance it can play in being a successful caregiver. Humor buddies won't be hard to find. They're the happy, sociable ones, with outgoing personalities and overflowing humor capacities, whose outlook on life is as contagious as a baby's smile.

The more you share with your humor buddies, the better you get at sharing things that are funny. As their humor rubs off on you, yours will rub off on them and you'll both be happier as a result. You'll build your self-esteem, hone your humor skills and become an even better caregiver.

My Strategy: _____

_____

■   BUILD A SUPPORT SYSTEM

"No one can whistle a symphony. It takes an orchestra to play it."
- Anonymous music critic.

It's a proven fact that people who have solid support systems survive the rigors of caregiving much better than those who don't.

A caregiver support system will provide a positive environment in which you can share your humor. But more importantly, the stress and frustration you experience in caregiving can be acknowledged, ventilated, clarified and redirected.

Track down caregiver support groups through newspapers, hospital social workers, community service agencies or other health-care professionals. Check the list of resources at the back of this book. It provides a number of places where you can begin your search for assistance.

You can join a formalized group of people who share a common concern over a specific illness or disability. Or you can be part of an informal network of family, friends and co-workers who are willing to help wherever they can. In either case, a support system will provide a smorgasbord of help, humor, escape, rewards, comfort, insight and strategies.

When you find a group that serves your needs, join it. Otherwise start one yourself. Attend the meetings and get involved in group activities. Draw on the knowledge and skill of your peers, and don't hesitate to offer your own suggestions.

Your introduction to a formal support group may be as frightening as an opening gig for a stand-up comic. Especially if you're meeting a group of people you've never seen before. They won't remain strangers for long, because everyone will understand and appreciate what everybody else is going through. Just knowing that someone else is facing problems similar to yours will renew your energy and give you a whole new outlook on life.

Support goes both ways. As you gain confidence and support from people in your group, you in turn can reach out to others who need to know that they are not alone.

"Give what you have. To some it may be better than you dare to think."
- Henry Wadsworth Longfellow, American poet.

My Strategy: _____

_____

■ COMMUNICATE

"Humor is often a way of communicating that allows things to be said that couldn't be said otherwise. My hope is that if we take humor more seriously, we'll be able to enjoy it more frequently." – Ralph Nader, American lawyer and consumer advocate.

Know what's involved in the way you communicate your humor. First there are the *words,* and sometimes they're not enough, even when you spend a lot of time and thought selecting them. The second part is made up of *vocal characteristics,* including the tone, emphasis and pitch of your voice. Last are the *nonverbal signals*—gestures, demeanor, expressions, physical appearance—which have little or nothing to do with words or voice. They represent what you're doing or how you look when you communicate.

Research has shown that the people you communicate with will take in 7 percent of your words, 38 percent of your vocal characteristics and *55 percent* of your nonverbal signals. This is particularly true of care receivers with dementia or Alzheimer's who communicate with feelings—not words.

As you can see, over half of what you're communicating when you're sharing your humor or expressing your concerns has nothing to do with what you say or how you say it. It has to do with your nonverbal signs. And since those signs reflect how you feel about what you're saying, they're going to determine how your care receiver and others are going to respond to you and your attempts at humor.

Use humor in your communication to relieve your pain, but be realistic in your comments if your problems are acute. No one will take you seriously if you let your sense of humor insulate you from the hard knocks and disappointments that are so often found in caregiving. Your nonverbal signals may cause greater stress if you make light of urgent needs or exaggerate them beyond belief.

Speak up when things bother you, but be diplomatic. Emphasize positive as well as negative points when expressing your concerns. If you hide your feelings or repress your cares under the cloak of feigned laughter, you'll erect communication barriers that will be hard to bring back down.

My Strategy: _____

_____

■ ADD HUMOR TO STRESS

"The sky is falling! The sky is falling!" - Chicken Little, fairy tale character.

Look for humor in those stressful, awkward or unpleasant situations that are often found in caregiving. If you can find something to laugh about, it will help discharge tension, reduce stress and chase away aggressive feelings that build up in every caregiver from time to time.

When you feel hurt or mad, take the initiative and use the magic of humor to provide an escape route where one is needed. Tell your potential combatant that your space ship is double parked, and much as you'd like to stay and argue, you really have other planets to visit. If done skillfully, your use of humor will relieve the stress and tension of a close encounter of the caregiving kind.

Make sure your humor lasts until another time. Whatever you use to break the tension, make it short and sweet so others will not forget what you said or did. If they talk about it later, it will help prevent another stress-provoking incident, and you will be remembered as a friend. The more of these humorous, stress-and-tension-breakers you can accumulate, the better you will be in handling caregiving situations that others might find difficult.

Sometimes it helps to ease the stress of caregiving by taking yourself out of a difficult situation. Use your imagination and visualize how the episode would play on stage or TV. Imagine how actors, comedians, politicians, or cartoon characters would handle it. Take a clue from your fantasy world, and assume the role of a humorous peacemaker. Even poor imitations of John Wayne or Ma

Kettle can break the ice and provide a lighthearted escape for everyone involved.

Add a little humor to stressful situations whenever you get a chance. It might seem incongruous, but if you didn't laugh at your misfortunes, you'd have to find other ways of surviving, and some of them can be a lot harder than coming up with a chuckle or two.

My Strategy: _____

_____

■   **TAKE HUMOR BREAKS**

"Time spent laughing is time spent with the gods." - Japanese proverb.

Stop, whenever you can during a stressful caregiving day, and take a humor break for 5 or 10 minutes. Retreat to your humortorium, or someplace like it, where you can be by yourself. Sit back, relax, refer to your humor journal or scrapbook and try a smile on for size.

Take a break not only from the tasks at hand, but also from your surroundings and the people with whom you are involved. If you think your days are too hectic for humor breaks, try to squeeze in some time in the morning before your care receiver gets up or after bedtime at night.

A humor break will put you into a world of your own for just a few minutes and let you forget work, caregiving and everything else that's weighing heavily on your nerves. It's like changing a baby's diaper. It doesn't solve the problem, but it does make things more comfortable for a while.

You may not be fortunate enough to work with or care for people who have a great sense of humor. Even if you do, you can't always count on them for a laugh every time you need a humor fix. It's better to take the initiative and do what you have to do to find respite. Set aside a special time of your own and organize your efforts to insure that your humor break is successful.

If possible, add to your *Dr. Seuss Journal,* if not daily, then weekly. Hopefully, your assortment of songs, jokes, stories, cartoons, personal experiences and/or recollections should generate some immediate giggles and brighten your day. Don't worry if no one else thinks your selections are funny. You want the notes that give *you* the laugh that refreshes when you need it most. Refine your collection as it grows and cull out items that have grown stale and timeworn.

Jot down key words about past experiences that tickled your funny bone. If you thought Victor Borge's concert on TV was a riot, write Victor Borge—as two of your keys words—on a card and keep the card in your pocket. Do the same with words like *prom, wedding, first date, circus,* or *Fourth of July parade.*

Refer to your key word card every time you take your humor break. Your key words will not only help you recall situations that made you laugh in the past, they may even help you get through a difficult caregiving situation in the present.

Don't discount the humor break as another caregiving gimmick. It's an essential component in the arsenal of caregiver survival tools. If you're feeling overwhelmed by the number of things you have to do, just think of it as driving two tons of canaries in a one-ton truck. The secret is to keep half of them in the air at all times.

My Strategy: _____

_____

This is the last of our strategies. Hopefully, as you went through them, others came to mind and you wrote them down. If you did, then you should have a good "starter list" of things that will help you discover the magic of humor in caregiving. All you need now is a plan of action to put those ideas into practice. You'll find one when you turn to the next section.

PLAN OF ACTION

☐ THE LAST LAP

"With humor not only do I feel more whole inside, and not only do I feel closer to those about me, but I also feel a quality of elevation, raising the realm of consciousness to a space that is larger than before...as for me, humor has more than comforted me through some difficult times. It has helped me make sense and meaning of my disability." - Arnold Beisser, graduate of Stanford University and its medical school, clinical professor of psychiatry at the University of California at Los Angeles, former national tennis champion, author of *Flying Without Wings*, and polio survivor.

Humor is a vital component of individual wellness for you and your care receiver. For you, the comic relief of laughing preserves your ability to function under stress. It increases your productivity and helps prevent caregiver burnout. Humor strengthens your perspective and dissipates panic, frustration and tension.

At the same time, your sense of humor will provide a warm and enlightening environment in which your care receiver can find relief from the disability or illness that demands your care. Your lighthearted approach will build trust, reduce the fear of unfamiliar pathways, and create a therapeutic relationship in which mental and physical distress can be softened.

You need two basic elements to discover and apply the magic of humor in caregiving:

- the ability to see the irony in the painful situations that often characterize the giving of care.

- a commitment to use that irony as a foundation for humor.

Here are five easy-to-apply strategies you can implement right now that will help you build on that foundation.

1. **Make Yourself Laugh:** Stick with those things that tickle your funny bone.

2. **Make a Friend Laugh:** Check out the stories, cartoons and one-liners that will make a good friend (with a well-developed sense of humor) laugh easily. The real test of your storytelling ability is this: your friend starts laughing just looking at you, even before you get to say anything.

3.   **Make Your Spouse or Relative Laugh:** You and your spouse or relative probably have very different interpretations of what is funny. If both of you find something amusing, you've narrowed your search considerably. Like you falling downstairs while warning your spouse not to.

4.   **Make Your Caregiver Support Group Laugh:** This is an audience that's doing many of the same things you are and sharing many of the same heartaches and pleasures. If you see them respond with a good-to-very-good chuckle, you know your material has got to be good. If you can make their eyes water, you're a pro.

5.   **Make Your Care Receiver Laugh:** Even some of your favorite bits of humor will fall flat on occasion. But the best ones should go over well in any situation and strike your care receiver as being funny. That's a mighty good indicator of the kind of material you need to stimulate your sense of humor and make your care receiver feel better.

Let this be a new beginning. Become a lighthearted caregiver and discover the magic of humor. The sooner you act, the sooner you'll start feeling better. You've had time to think about it. Now it's time to act.

"There are enough tragedies in life; we have to have some laughs."
- Steve Allen, American humorist.

AVAILABLE RESOURCES

It would be impossible to provide an up-to-date list of available caregiving resources for every area of the country. Or for that matter, other countries besides the United States where caregivers are found. What is provided here is a generic list of people, agencies and organizations that can provide help when the need arises.

Use this list as an entry to your phone book, community service agency or support group and build a list of your own. Just be sure to share it with the next caregiver you meet. There is no one who needs help more than one who has nowhere to turn.

Hospitals
Senior centers
Support groups
Legal aid services
State units on aging
Volunteer programs
Ombudsman services
In-house respite care
Home chore services
Home health services
Home-delivered meals
Housekeeping services
Area agencies on aging
Veteran's affairs offices
Senior citizen's services
Adult day care programs
Out-of-home respite care
County extension services
Caregiver resource centers

Community health services
County public health nurses
Social security district offices
Economic assistance agencies
State human services agencies
County human service agencies
Illness and disability associations
Information and referral agencies
Illness and disability treatment centers
Mental health and counseling agencies
Social service agencies sponsored by governmental bodies
Social service agencies affiliated with a church or association

There are many agencies that provide support in specialized areas dealing with diseases like Alzheimer's, Parkinson's, stroke or diabetes. Many others offer help to people who have ailments related to parts of the body such as brain, heart, lungs or kidneys.

You might start by calling the United Way, the National Council on Aging, the American Association of Retired Persons or the Eldercare Information and Referral Service at 1-800-677-1116.

The thing to remember is that *you are not alone.* There are millions of people all over the world who understand your problems and are willing to help.

INDEX

NOTES

NOTES

NOTES

ABOUT THE AUTHOR

James R. Sherman is the author and publisher of 20 books, including the national bestseller, *Stop Procrastinating—DO IT!*, which has sold over 350,000 copies. His books have been reproduced on cassette tape, marketed worldwide, and translated into Chinese, French, German, Hungarian, Japanese, Polish and Spanish. Dr. Sherman has appeared on the NBC TODAY show as well as on regional and local radio and television programs. His self–help articles have appeared in national, regional, and local publications. His lively and entertaining talks about success, procrastination, humor and caregiving have rounded out his publishing career.

Born and raised in southwestern Minnesota, Dr. Sherman received his bachelor's and master's degrees from the University of Colorado and his doctorate from the University of Northern Colorado. Following positions as Assistant Professor of Educational Psychology at the University of Minnesota and Assistant Chancellor of the Minnesota Community College System, Jim spent seven years as a management consultant to colleges and universities across the country. He established Pathway Books in 1979 and has devoted full time to his writing, speaking, and publishing efforts ever since. He does much of his writing at his cabin adjacent to the Boundary Waters Canoe Area Wilderness in northern Minnesota.

He now brings his extensive caregiving experience to his writing in a new 12–book, self–help series for caregivers.

ABOUT THE SENIOR EDITOR

Merlene Sherman completed graduate studies in nursing home and hospital administration at the University of Minnesota and has worked in geriatrics for 20 years. She worked extensively with caregivers while developing and directing two adult daycare programs in Minneapolis.

Merlene is internationally known for her programs in workplace wellness and is the author of two health promotion books, *Wellness in the Workplace* and *Health Strategies for Working Women*. More recently, she and her husband Jim have been involved in producing the Caregiver Survival Series and speaking at conferences and seminars. Their focus has been on caregivers and the professionals who serve them.

For over 13 years Merlene and Jim were caregivers to both sets of parents, now deceased. They have three adult sons and now enjoy playing with, doting upon, and overfeeding their grandchildren.

THE CAREGIVER SURVIVAL SERIES

Preventing Caregiver Burnout

Caregivers who work long, hard hours under constant emotional pressure can very easily lose their motivation and commitment to caregiving. This dynamic book responds to that threat by describing what burnout is, what causes it, and what effect it can have on a caregiver's vitality. Best of all, it presents an extensive list of easy–to–follow procedures for preventing burnout and maintaining an optimistic outlook toward caregiving.

Creative Caregiving

This book inspires caregivers to develop creative ways of relieving the most maddening aspects of caregiving. It provides a wealth of innovative techniques that show caregivers how to work smarter, not harder, and make the most of precious free time. Once they read this book, caregivers will wonder how they ever got along without it.

Positive Caregiver Attitudes

A "must" book for any caregiver whose back is against the wall. It's loaded with down–to–earth strategies for developing and maintaining positive attitudes toward care receivers, caregiving, and life in general. The book identifies the source of negative feelings and illustrates the destructive effect negative attitudes can produce if left unresolved. It provides a vital safeguard for any caregiving relationship.

The Magic of Humor in Caregiving

This resourceful book provides tremendous benefits and tickles funny bones at the same time. It clearly explains the well-established healing benefits of laughter in reducing stress and tension. And without being disrespectful of the conditions that bring caregivers and care receivers together, the book shows how playfulness can be used to increase personal effectiveness, promote wellness and lighten the impact of one of life's misfortunes. It helps caregivers see caregiving in a new and refreshing ways and leaves no doubt that laughter is often the best medicine that caregivers can use.

The Caregiver's Guide to Problem Solving

This eye–opening book helps caregivers identify problems, determine their root causes, explore alternative strategies, make realistic choices, and implement effective solutions to caregiving problems. It's an indispensable tool that takes the guesswork out of day–to–day decision making and makes the hard job of caregiving much easier. No caregiver should be without it.

Conquering Caregiver Fears

This dynamite book pinpoints the sources of fear, anxiety, guilt, and depression, and tells why they exist. It outfits caregivers with surefire methods for controlling anxiety, building courage, and maintaining the self–confidence they need to conquer the destructive forces that often accompany and threaten caregiving. This is a no–nonsense manual that will stand up under years of repeated use.

Strengthening the Caregiver Family

Holding a family together and dealing with interpersonal conflicts is a challenge for many caregivers. This timely book outlines the sources of family conflict, then puts forth an ample supply of time–tested solutions for building and maintaining family harmony. It empowers caregivers to tackle unmet needs, sibling rivalries, generational differences, caregiving role disputes and other difficulties with confidence and conviction.

Love, Companionship and Caregiving

This revealing book helps caregivers recognize the physical and emotional challenges that interfere with normal expressions of love, affection, and companionship. Its down–to–earth strategies help caregivers deal with the physical and emotional burdens that frequently accompany caregiving. Readers gain a clear perspective on how to recognize problems, overcome obstacles, and meet basic personal needs while in a caregiving relationship. Creative suggestions tell how to maintain tender, intimate relationships and turn difficult moments into priceless memories.

Health Strategies for Active Caregivers

A made–to–order book that highlights the special health and fitness needs of caregivers and shows how those needs can be satisfied within the caregiving environment. It provides detailed instructions for staying in excellent condition while meeting the unrelenting demands of the caregiver role. Wellness strategies for nutrition, exercise, sleep, and stress reduction show caregivers how to maintain a healthy lifestyle.

The Caregiver's Need for People

This candid book focuses on the caregiver's need for extensive human interaction, not just with the care receiver, but with family, friends, health care professionals, and other caregivers. It stresses the importance of making new friends and keeping existing friendships intact. The book provides an ample supply of techniques for enhancing social contacts and opportunities. This book is standard equipment for anyone who is involved in an activity that is as people–intensive as caregiving.

The Caregiver's Planning Guide

Caregivers, in almost every case, soon discover that they must respond quickly and effectively to the never–ending demands of an unpredictable future. This superb planning guide helps clarify the caregivers present position, helps them determine where they want to be in the future, and shows them what they have to do to get there. It provides an abundance of time–proven procedures for developing workable plans for taking the drudgery out of caregiving.

Financial Fitness for Caregivers

This user–friendly book provides an in–depth look at the financial demands that often overwhelm unsuspecting caregivers. It's loaded with cost–effective suggestions for alleviating financial stress, discovering new sources of funds and meeting special caregiving needs. Every caregiver who has had to face the continuous rise in health–care costs will find this book to be an effective weapon against financial worries.

HOW TO ORDER

Now you can build a library of outstanding self-help books for caregivers with no hassle and at an unbelievably low price.

The subject matter of the 12 books in the *Caregiver Survival Series* covers some of the major concerns of millions of people just like you. The books give you easy-to-understand explanations of why you're having problems. They also give you clear, concise guidelines for eliminating those problems and turning your life as a caregiver into a compelling and rewarding experience.

The books are easy to come by. Just call or fax us at 612-377-1521 or make a copy of the order form on the next page and send it to our Golden Valley address. Tell us how many copies you want of each title, add 6.5% for Minnesota sales tax and an appropriate amount for shipping, and include your check or money order. We'll have your books in the mail within 24-48 hours. If you order more than 10 books, we'll bill you for the actual shipping costs.

The books in the *Caregiver Survival Series* are guaranteed to make you a better caregiver. If—for any reason—you're not satisfied, send your books back, and you'll get an immediate refund. We'll still keep your name on our mailing list so you won't miss out on any news about future books in the series.

ORDER FORM

Title	Price	No.		Cost
Preventing Caregiver Burnout	$ 7.95 x		=	$ _____
Creative Caregiving	$ 7.95 x		=	$ _____
Positive Caregiver Attitudes	$ 7.95 x		=	$ _____
The Magic of Humor in Caregiving	$ 7.95 x		=	$ _____
The Caregiver's Guide to Problem Solving	$ 7.95 x		=	$ _____
Conquering Caregiver Fears	$ 7.95 x		=	$ _____
Strengthening the Caregiver Family	$ 7.95 x		=	$ _____
Love, Compassion, and Caregiving	$ 7.95 x		=	$ _____
Health Strategies for Active Caregivers	$ 7.95 x		=	$ _____
The Caregiver's Need for People	$ 7.95 x		=	$ _____
The Caregiver's Planning Guide	$ 7.95 x		=	$ _____
Financial Fitness for Caregivers	$ 7.95 x		=	$ _____

Shipping Charges   Subtotal $ _____

1 copy   = $1.50   6.5% MN sales tax $ _____
2–5 copies   = $ 2.00
6-10 copies = $ 2.50   Shipping charges $ _____
10+ copies   = actual

                                    NET DUE $ _____

* These four books are currently available. The remaining books in the series will be completed in 1996 and 1997.

SHIP TO (Please type or print clearly)

NAME: _____

ADDRESS: _____

_____

CITY/STATE/ZIP: _____

PHONE: _____ DATE: _____

━━

BILL TO (If different from above)

NAME: _____

ADDRESS: _____

_____

CITY/STATE/ZIP: _____

PHONE: _____ DATE: _____

Pathway Books
700 Parkview Terrace
Golden Valley, MN 55416
(612) 377–1521